Spanish Flu 1918, Deadlier Than Covid-19

The 1918 H1N1 flu pandemic killed an estimated 50 million people worldwide, including an estimated 675,000 people in the United States. The virus' unique severity puzzled researchers for decades, and prompted several questions. These questions drove an expert group of researchers and virus hunters to search for the lost 1918 virus, sequence its genome, and recreate the virus in a highly safe and regulated laboratory setting at CDC.

The epidemic's origin is unclear. It was found in March 1918 among American troops in Kansas. Infected military convoys would then spread throughout Europe.
First in spring 1918, then two more severe waves due to viral alterations making it more aggressive.
(H1N1), the same virus that produced the 2009 pandemic (which killed 18.500 according to the OMS and over 200.000 by two post-mortem estimations). Although they are believed to be direct or indirect ancestors of the 1918 virus, infectious A-type viruses are considerably less severe.
Aside from the elderly and tiny kids, the Spanish flu mostly affected young people. Its target market was 20-40 years olds.
The grippal virus caused severe respiratory blockages in birds, leading to death. War facilitated viral transmission, although wounds and privations reduced immune defences, explaining the severity of the pandemic.

The epidemic's cost is unknown. It was formerly estimated as nearly 21 million. Recent estimates put the global infection rate at one-third, with at least half a million fatalities.

In 2002, Niall Johnson and Juergen Mueller calculated the epidemic's "true bilan" at 100 million.

The epidemic has hit many countries. Despite strict quarantine, Australia is among the least impacted.

The SDN established the Health Committee and the Organization of Hygiene in 1922, forerunners of the WHO (OMS).

Famous casualties of the Flu pandemic included Egon Schiele, Guillaume Apollinaire, and Edmond Rostand.

During the month of September, 1918, a highly infectious and lethal sickness spread like wildfire over the United States. It was a virulent pandemic, featuring many of the symptoms of influenza, as well as a deadly lung disease Many were in the dark about the condition, or about how to deal with it, and both the medical community and public health organizations were scrambling to come up with an answer.

Although new measures may have been instituted to mitigate the spread of the disease, the population at large failed to comprehend the extent of the threat they were facing.

This was definitely a disturbing discovery, for all across the country, a large number of people had come together through the Red Cross and other well-known and efficient organizations to fight disease and prevent suffering and death, and yet we were struck with a disastrous plague that killed more people in the United States than the bombs and poison gas used by the enemy overseas in the Great War.

Folks receiving data from the Federal Census Bureau told the Federal Census Bureau that between September 9 and November 9, there were a total of 82,306

Spanish Flu 1918, Deadlier Than Covid-19

deaths related to the disease. In the same timeframe, throughout the same communities, the flu and pneumonia normally results in 4,000 deaths.

Reports began coming in around the beginning of October that the disease was being reported in nearly all of the U.S. states, ranging from eastern Massachusetts in the east to northern California in the west and from the southern part of Florida in the south-east to the northern half of Washington in the north-west. During a twenty-four-hour period, at least 14,000 cases were reported throughout the military camps of the country to the office of the Surgeon General of the Army.

These Census Bureau statistics indicate that, up until January 4, 1919, a total of 115,258 deaths occurred as a result of the fatal disease in the United States. The Actuarial Society of America's findings, however, indicate that 450,000 deaths occurred in the United States during the autumn and early winter of 1918 due to this pandemic disease, which struck mostly infants and working-age adults. Males had a higher mortality rate, but it was due to sickness, not aging, whereas the largest mortality caused by the disease was found among persons who made their living wage or more—especially those in the lowest economic stratum.

The disease's origin or source remained unknown. Some analysts considered it just a centuries-old problem that emerged from time to time with sporadic outbursts of violence occurring regularly. Other experts proposed a sort of pneumonic plague that has been raging in China for several years, called China and its bordering Asian countries an enormous reservoir of infection.

It is a historical fact that, in the first six or seven years of the twentieth century, an estimated 200,000 coolies were brought from China, where a massive epidemic of the pneumonic plague had broken out, to France, where they worked as laborers and also unwittingly brought the bacteria that caused the pneumonic plague. As a result of being seized by the Germans in the spring of 1918, there is a widely held belief that the disease was quite devastating in its virulence in the German army at that time.

Despite the German submarines, some press writers have stated that the disease arrived in the country, and after it was known that it was sweeping through

Europe like a plague of the Middle Ages, it was called by many specialists a by-product of World War One.

The ways in which the pandemic appeared in various countries suggest that the disease's germs were spread there by the winds. When this notion was put forth, it was claimed that deadly vapors had drifted with the winds, spreading the pandemic throughout Europe, Asia, Africa, and the Americas.

Even in the north, the disease had deadly consequences even in lonely Labrador, the "silent North" of the Western Hemisphere, where ice-floes from farther north fill every harbor on the rock-bound coast; where giant icebergs, miles in length, mountains in height, and acres in extent, obstruct the path of ships and steamers.

This applies to Labrador's northern coastline, which spans 8 degrees of latitude, where no doctor, no nurse, no hospital, and no dispensary are to be found. Most Eskimos, Indians, Germans, and Brits fell victim to the dreadful calamity, which moved quickly from place to place. Civil single settlement was abandoned—all the corpses unburied, and being consumed by starving dogs. This is the horrifying account that emerged out of the "Silent North"— the world's scariest, bloodiest and most horrible illness and death to bear witness to.

The affliction first appeared in Germany and was named "Spanische Influenza" by its spread to Spain. It is not correct to call this disease an "epidemic", but this is one of the first epidemics of influenza that Spain has ever encountered, so the name has stayed. In the United States, per some slangologists, this sickness was known as "the flu," from which we get the word "influenza."

This terrible epidemic, which struck the state of Pennsylvania just prior to the start of World War One, first appeared in widely dispersed locations in the middle of September, 1918. The Commonwealth of Massachusetts on October 1 issued administrative orders to cease all public assemblies, burial services, bar businesses, and liquor stores, in addition to instructing the shutting of all motion picture houses, theaters, and entertainment places. It was left to the discretion of local governments to decide whether to close schools, churches, and Sunday schools. Additionally, the Department published proclamations and pleas encouraging everyone to contribute to the success of fighting the epidemic.

Spanish Flu 1918, Deadlier Than Covid-19

Early on October 3, October 4, and October 5, the State Department of Health directives and pleas were promptly and happily obeyed. However, on the first day of the spread of the disease, only twenty cases were reported.

The Wyoming Valley Chapter of the Red Cross, realizing that military medical personnel and registered nurses are in short supply, recently made an appeal on October 3 to find qualified female nurses and women with some nursing experience to register with the Chapter.

The following guidelines and directions are contained in a circular letter sent on October 8, 1914, by the Commissioner of Health of Pennsylvania to the Department of Health and other physicians in the state with a mandate to combat the Influenza Epidemic:

The Commonwealth's Governor, Commissioner of Health, and Advisory Board of the Pennsylvania Department of Health have all come to the conclusion that, given the current influenza pandemic, the use of the organization at hand, along with all available organizations, must be the highest priority in order to save the lives of our people. Subsequently, following thorough deliberation, the following courses of action have been adopted:

It is absolutely essential that the federal Department of Health exert complete control over the program and assume complete responsibility.

The formation of nineteen Epidemic Emergency Districts, each headed by a Commissioner of Health with direct authority from the Commissioner of Health, who transmits his instructions to the Epidemic Emergency Corps and delivers them to those who answer the call to assist with all possible under the direction.

The Adjutant General has made available to us for the installation of emergency hospitals, the supply of goods, the protection of property, and the maintenance of discipline all of the resources and assets of his department.

Aid requests from impacted populations should be submitted to the local Epidemic Emergency District Physician. This is any cry for aid from doctors, nurses, or other caregivers. To address any such requests as promptly as possible, the Department will do every effort. In these instances, nevertheless, they should be obtained as close to the assignment as possible.

All employees should use protective masks.

influenza and pneumonia are treated

Dr. Charles H. Miner of Wilkes-Barre, who had been the County Medical Inspector of the state Department of Health for Luzerne County for ten years, was named the supervisor of District No. 5 on October 8th, when the acting commissioner of health (Dr. B. Franklin Royer) appointed him.

In the morning, the Acting Commissioner of Pennsylvania phoned the County Medical Inspector in Wilkes-Barre, Pennsylvania, and asked him to have Wilkes-Barre Major General C. B. Dougherty contacted the State Surgeon in Harrisburg so the two of them could develop and organize plans for properly handling the situation in the 5th District.

To respond to the call for their services, the military generals of the Army Medical Department, namely General Daugherty, and the County Medical Inspector worked rapidly to determine that due to the fact that the regular and permanent hospitals located in the 5th District were overflowing with influenza and pneumonia patients, and that each day new cases were being reported in each of the communities, that several emergency hospitals would have to be established and equipped.

In light of the additional 60 new cases of influenza, the county medical inspector decided to establish an emergency hospital in Wilkes-Barragher (where on October 8, there were 60 new cases), and the armory of the 9th Regiment, National Guard of Pennsylvania, located on South Main Street, was selected for the task.

The armory, which had been the headquarters of the 2d Infantry, Pennsylvania Reserve Militia (Col. S. E. W. Eyer in charge), had been in use for some time.

Colonel Eyer turned over the armory to the Department of Health on October 8, and Daugherty, under his supervision, had the building cleaned to the top and bottom by the end of the day. Once the Shepherd Construction Company of Wilkes-Barre had started the construction of four wards on the drill floor of the armory, construction of the fourth ward commenced on the drill floor of the armory.

Each of these wards had an area of 2,127 feet by 10 feet, and each had a corresponding height of 10 feet. Hemlock studding covered with beaver board was used to form the partitions. Every ward contained fifteen cots, giving each patient adequate room to breathe. In order to make it easier for nurses and attendants to give appropriate care and attention to hospital patients, considerable plumbing work had to be done. When the plumbing work was finished, it had cost $605.49. The armory does not have enough lighting facilities, to put it simply. The wiring and lights throughout the entire structure had to be installed, which cost $190.

As it turned out, this setup was only able to house sixty patients, but as it became apparent that the hospital needed more space, four more wards of the same dimensions and materials were built. The overall capacity of these eight wards, when finished, was 120 beds. Out of these eight wards, six were assigned to patients who were hospitalized, one was reserved for patients with pneumonia in the last stages, and one was designated for patients recovering from pneumonia.

A spacious and comfortable dining room was built into the basement of the armory; moreover, a sanitary kitchen was painted white, and gas stoves were connected to it while refrigerators were added a separate diet kitchen was set up on the main level of the armory, making it easy for students and guests to get a bite to eat.

General Daugherty was asked to be present on the evening of October 9, and Hayden Williams, the Chamber of Commerce's Secretary, was also appointed to handle the evening's clerical duties.

The County Medical Inspector spent a lot of time explaining how preparations were being made for the opening of the Armory Emergency Hospital in

Wilkes-Barre. He made the following statement: He had divided the 5th District into five sub-districts. It was proposed that committees be formed to handle the auto industry, food, pharmaceuticals, and general hospital supplies.

In 1867, General Daugherty gave an account of the serious conditions in the 3rd Congressional District and adjacent areas in the 5th Congressional District, where he testified to Congress. During the presentation given by Dr. Underwood and Miss Tinsley, information on the conditions in Exeter, Luzerne County, where there were around 300 cases, was discussed. 182 instances were reported in 62 homes; 98 patients were convalescing; 10 families were in desperate need of assistance; and a unique need exists for women to assist with the household chores of families who are affected by the outbreak.

The sanitary conditions were severe, as well as a dearth of nurses, and the newly renovated high school in Wanamie was now being used as an emergency hospital.

Dr. G. A. Clark, the city health official for Wilkes-Barre, announced that there had been around 200 documented cases of the sickness, and that the city would be held responsible for the cost of combating it.

According to Dr. Lake, there were 36 cases in Kingston, and 40 in Edwardsville, and two or three deaths occurred as a result. Seven instances of mad cow disease were found in one home in Edwardsville. Toby's Creek, which had never been cleaned, may aid tremendously if placed in hygienic condition.

Catawissa's health issues required a hospital but couldn't be met with the number of nurses who were available. The disease has now been contracted by six individuals in that location, and it appears to be spreading. He reported that the saloons in Centralia were wide open and that the school-houses in Bloomsburg were being turned into emergency hospitals.

Conyngham, the Red Cross representative from the Wyoming Valley Chapter, announced that his chapter did not have money to hire nurses, but that his people were prepared to do anything they could to help the patients in the community.

Spanish Flu 1918, Deadlier Than Covid-19

Dr. Mengel, the Chief Surgeon for the Lehigh Valley Coal Company, recommended that school teachers may be used to help care for the sick in the community, and the nurses who worked there were made available to the public.

As one of the Commissioners of Luzerne County, Mr. McLaughlin made assurances that the county would offer any aid feasible to help terminate the outbreak.

In cooperation with the employees of the Wilkes-Barre Chamber of Commerce, the Secretary took care of all the work that came with the campaign. Dr. Charles Long proposed that a request be made to the Board of Directors of the Central Poor District of Luzerne County for financial and other help.

County Fuel Administrator Anthony Campbell addressed the deteriorating conditions in the mining business and mentioned that anthracite coal output was suffering due to the epidemic. Following the motion of Mr. Campbell, it was then unanimously agreed that those hospitals whose status as an emergency hospital had been decided upon by the County Medical Inspector be established, as well as those in charge of the work connected with combating the influenza-pneumonia scourge asking for funding from the Board of Directors of the Central Poor District, county officials, and municipal officers in the 5th District for any and all expenses they may incur.

After the meeting was adjourned, and it was publicized in the press within a day or two thereafter, the County Medical Inspector made the following announcement:

Convention General Committee:

To supervise all hospitals To secure various ways and means, including financial aid from various towns, and give fiscal support from various governmental entities. The Treasurer of the General Committee will hold all money donated, barring state funds. No expenditures may be made without prior approval from the General Committee and its Chairman.

Emergency Room Management Team

In responsibility for the development of emergency hospitals, this committee will be responsible for everything from financial planning to the day-to-day operation of the facilities.

The following physicians from Wilkes-Barre, Pittston, Kingston, Berwick, Plymouth, Nanticoke, and Bloomsburg are all planning to attend this year's annual meeting: Dr. S. P. Mengel of Wilkes-Barre, Chairman; Drs. Lewis H. Taylor, W. S. Stewart, and L. A. Sheridan of Wilkes-Barre; Dr. Cohen of Berwick, Dr. H. B. Wilcox of Kingston, Dr. H. Whitney of Plymouth, Dr. H. J. Lenahan of Pittston, Dr. Jesse Hughes of Nanticoke, Dr. J. H. Bruner of Bloomsburg, and Dr. Walter Lathrop.

to assist with the canteen expenses

Additionally, the committee shall offer the preparation of food for distribution to outpatients and the provision of the same for delivery to patients at their homes.

This Relief Committee will be composed of the women of the Red Cross Canteen Service, with Mrs. E. Birney Carr as Chairman.

This committee, directed by the Emergency Hospital Committee, has responsibility for maintaining the hospital's sanitary environment and for disposing of garbage.

Staff members at the Armory Hospital provide direct aid to the Emergency Hospital Superintendent and assume assignments from time to time, which is determined by the Emergency Hospital Committee Chairman.

The Committee on Motor Transportation

This committee oversees the motor transportation required for transporting patients and nurses from hospitals to their homes and vice versa. Men will be formed under this committee into a sub-committee that will coordinate the transport of food to individual homes.

Committee that aids nurses

This committee is responsible for the recruitment and selection of all of the trained nurses, Red Cross nurses, and volunteer nurses, as well as the recruitment of visiting nurses for the emergency hospitals and homes. Association of convenience store operators

To assist the hospitals in times of emergencies, this committee will organize the pharmacy stores and make sure that the pharmacies have in stock medicines and medical items that will be required. Second, to reserve and maintain a supply of pharmaceuticals and medical supplies for the hospital in case of an emergency.

Edward H. White, lieutenant, and Henry W. Merritt are also on the board of directors.

Luzerne County Co-operation Committee.

To aid and collaborate in every way to prevent the spread of the disease, the municipal governments and the Boards of Health in their respective areas have established a house-to-house census committee and report all cases of illness to the Chairman of the General Committee. The meeting will be under the control of the General Committee, but the other committees may convene as well. Community Captains should report to their Community Chairmen and those Chairmen should then inform their District Chairmen. Those District Chairmen then inform the General Chairman of the Coöperation Committee of what they learn each day. The last thing to be reported to Dr. Miner about the State Department of Health's actions is what happened yesterday.

The county commissioners from Luzerne County.

Boroughs and hamlets are in the boroughs and townships of Courtdale, Dallas, Dorranceton, Exeter, Forty Fort, Kingston, Luzerne, Pringle, Shavertown, Swoyersville, Trucksville, West Pittston, Wyoming, and West Wyoming.

District No. 2, which comprises the boroughs of Edwardsville, Larksville, Plymouth, and Shickshinny, as well as the townships of Fairmount, Hunlock, Huntington, Jackson, Lake, Lehman, Plymouth, Ross, Salem, and Union, is located in western Schuylkill County.

Spanish Flu 1918, Deadlier Than Covid-19

District No. 3, which covers the city and townships of Pittston and Avoca, as well as the boroughs of Dupont, Duryea, and Hughestown, is an accurate representation of the region's current makeup.

District No. 4 is made up of the boroughs of Laflin, Miner's Mills, Parsons, and Yatesville, as well as the townships of Jenkins and Plains.

The five boroughs of Ashley, Laurel Run, Nuangola, Sugar Notch, and Warrior Run, as well as the townships of Wilkes-Barre, Fairview, Bear Creek, Buck, Wright, Slocum, and Denison comprise District No. 5.

District No. 6, comprises the borough of Nanticoke, the village of Macanaqua, the borough and township of Nescopeck, and the townships of Conyngham, Dorrance, Hollenback, Newport, and Slocum.

The city of Hazleton and all terrain that is contiguous to it make up District No. 7.

Following are the regulations on how community groups are to be operated and the guidelines for each unit of a community organization:

The chair of the community.

As Chairman of the Executive Committee, shall perform all management and operational tasks and have complete responsibility for each unit. Get daily reports from all subordinates, and make reports to the District Chairman.

"an executive committee

It is agreed that an employee shall never be required to work without direct supervision from the Community Chairman. This committee will assist the Community Chairman in implementing all of the rules and regulations.

"Number three: secretary.

This involves the person being on duty at the Emergency Station all the time. Collect and organize all case information, as well as any other information that is requested. As a supervisor, prepare a daily report for the community

chairman, and at the same time, handle all calls for nurses, canteen service, and medical treatment. Involve a school instructor if it is desired that the Secretary have assistance.
"in case of an emergency

Conveniently placed in the heart of the city. Secretary and other officials can use it for a telephone. Be open for business during normal business hours.

Every group has a captain.

Each community will have a Captain under the guidance of the Community Chairman and Executive Committee. To increase the number of captains for an abnormally lengthy street, it must be noted in the street's profile. Each day, the captain of each street will tour their community and will inform the Community Chairman, the Chairman of the Local Emergency Response Team, and the Secretary at the Local Emergency Station about new cases, fatalities, and discharged cases. Captains will also be attentive to the health and general well-being of the passengers and will be there to help them if conditions or illness spreads on board. Captain's reports include any medical cases and those that require medical attention.

The nursing bureau has 6 agents.

emergency medical personnel who supervise the program's implementation Every woman who volunteers as a nurse or nurse's helper should maintain a record in this section. This bureau should also provide nurses' gowns and masks to help them at the house of the sick when they are caring for the sick.

There is a service called "Canteen Service" that supplies meals to the ailing people where it is required. The users of this service should be mindful that it can be misused. In order to increase the volume of calls being answered, the Canteen should be constructed, preferably in a church kitchen, and broth or soup should be produced and provided in jars or pails to the doors of the homes from which the phone rings.

Automobile service is eight.

As well as doing regular service rounds to the hospital and clinic, take one car or truck per day to service machinery at the canteen and other locations to transport nurses and physicians to the residences of patients when necessary. The publicity bureau is 9.

a job where you assume responsibility for making sure the distribution of pamphlets in multiple languages, spreading general information, and publicizing regulation enforcement happens

"LEGAL STRUCTURE.

This community organization wants everyone to know the gravity of the problem, and they've placed responsibility on each individual to enforce every rule.

After the conditions are right, it is easier to prevent an epidemic than to try to contain one when it is already underway.

Just tell individuals you are concerned about their well-being but that you must also insist that they don't expose themselves to sickness or spread it.

Don't allow the public to gather in groups of three or more on the streets, in stores, or anywhere.

Neither should there be any public funerals, and for funerals, an officer from the police or the health department should be present to ensure that the law is being enforced.

The saying, "Safety First," shall be the guiding principle for all people.

Do not open schools or churches unless necessary.

Pursuant to the resolution adopted at the Chamber of Commerce meeting on October 9, which is mentioned above, Dr. Miner ordered the following new emergency hospitals to be established: In addition to the three hospitals that have already been set up at Wanamie and the Armory in Wilkes-Barre,

Spanish Flu 1918, Deadlier Than Covid-19

Pennsylvania, these locations are all located at the following: Catawissa, Exeter, Hazleton, Dupont, Nanticoke, and Plains.

All the hospitals located in the 5th District during that time were permanent, or regular, facilities: Wilkes-Barre City Hospital, Mercy Hospital, Wyoming Valley Homeopathic Hospital, and Riverside Hospital in Wilkes-Barre; Nesbitt West Side Hospital, Dorrance; Pittston Hospital, Pittston; Berwick Hospital, Berwick; Columbia County State Hospital of the Middle Coal Field Hospital, Hazleton; and Nanticoke State Hospital.

The first hospital specifically set up to care for victims of emergencies opened on October 10, in the Wanamie Central High School building, with Dr. William H. Corrigan in charge and Miss Emily G. Jones as the hospital's head nurse. In order to begin treating the sick patients in Catawissa's emergency hospital, Dr. S. B. Arment, the doctor in charge, and Miss Hannah C. Breisch, the head nurse, were all inaugurated on the same day. The newly opened third emergency hospital in Exeter, which began accepting patients on October 11, was headed by Dr. James Dixon, who was assisted by Jessie Cunningham and Ernest W. Hogg, Graduate Nurses.

When New York City Health Commissioner Royal S. Copeland transferred him to Wilkes-Barre, Pennsylvania, in the late 1930s, Dr. Elmer L. Hinman was dispatched to the County Medical Inspector's office to help Dr. Corrigan.

At that time, it was expected that at least 1,000 people had influenza and pneumonia, of which several hundred more had not yet been counted. Due to a lack of space and nurses, the Wilkes-Barre City Hospital declined taking any additional patients. Because so many nurses and doctors are overtaxed, conditions in Newport Township and Hazleton, as well as throughout the area, are very terrible.

A conference of the chairmen of several committees and division chairmen was conducted at the Chamber of Commerce on October 12th to determine whether or not to secure trucks to provide daily food delivery to the homes of the sick, where this was needed. Thus, both Percy A. Brown and Frank F. Matheson contributed vehicles in order to use them in this instance. Mrs. P. J. Higgins of Wilkes-Barre has been suggested as a cook for the Armory canteen. This person should be granted free rein to make all the arrangements, though the Canteen Committee retains control.

According to Dr. Mengel, a telegraph be sent to the appropriate authorities in Washington to let them know that they should leave this area before the outbreak of the epidemic, because all Red Cross nurses in the area will be affected. Reports from General Dougherty stated that he had contacted the Hon. A. Mitchell Palmer, as well as other Washington, D.C. officials, and had been guaranteed that ten army surgeons would be dispatched here from Camp Crane, Allentown, Pennsylvania.

After returning from the Boston area, where he had helped combat the epidemic, Dr. S. M. Wolfe described the different structured tactics and plans employed to control the sickness in that area.

After being voted to the Luzerne County National Bank's cashier position, Mr. William J. Ruff was subsequently chosen the county treasurer for the general committee.

After this meeting was adjourned, General Dougherty sent a telegram to Major General Rupert Blue, Surgeon General, U.S.A., and Dr. H. A. Garfield, the U.S. Fuel Administrator, along with the following message:

"This means that on Tuesday, October 15, four Red Cross nurses have been ordered to return to duty since they've been mobilized: Edith Evans, Elsie Banker, and Lena Krum from Wilkes-Barre; Hazel Smith from Tunkhannock; and Bessie Evans from Kingston. Due to the severity of the influenza outbreak in Wyoming Valley, and the shortage of nurses, I'm asking you to direct all of the nurses who are here to continue to help fight the infection by remaining at the emergency hospitals that are being established in order to save lives. I have great faith that you will see the value in this appeal. We're about to run out of both doctors and nurses, as well. An abundance of physicians and nurses is available for us to employ."

General Dougherty gave a report at the General Committee meeting on Tuesday, October 15th in the auditorium of the Chamber of Commerce, where conditions in Shamokin and Minersville (in the 3rd District) had risen to around 4,000

Spanish Flu 1918, Deadlier Than Covid-19

instances of "flu". Col. Eyer announced that the Armory Armory Hospital would be prepared to receive patients by noon the next day.

While speaking at a church service in Georgetown, St. Joseph's R.C. The Rev. John J. McCabe indicated that there were approximately 80 people infected with the disease in Wilkes-Barre Township. In Newport Township and nearby, there were roughly 585 instances, and Richard Sheridan put the number at around 200.

The chairman, Mr. McCabe, moved that Dr. C. H. Miner, the Reverend Mr. Jedlicka, and Dr. E. L. Meyers was appointed to a committee to meet with the Luzerne County Controller and Commissioners, as well as the Directors of the Central Poor District, and endeavor to obtain funding for fighting the outbreak. Controller Hendershot announced that he will work with the General Committee to help achieve the goals of the organization. Secretary of the Central District Board of Poor Management, James L. Reilly, commented that he was convinced the Board of Poor Management will collaborate with the Committee.

As a further extension of the free use of the ambulances of the Kingston Coal Company, Frederick E. Zerbey, Superintendent of the Kingston Coal Company, then volunteered to send those ambulances to ferry West Side patients across the river.

When asked about paying for all the costs of fighting the pandemic, such as health care, doctors, nurses, tents, cots, blankets, sheets, and everything else, General Dougherty said that everything would have to be paid for from money obtained from another source.

On October 16, the Hazleton Emergency Hospital (also known as the Hazleton Military Hospital) opened in the former St. Gabriel's High School building, Hazleton, with Lieutenant J. A. M. Aspy, the hospital's physician in charge, and Miss Ruth B. Rae, the Department of Health Graduate Nurse as the chief nurse. The Mother Superior of St. Gabriel's was a licensed nurse, and later in the movie, she became infected with the "flu" and was relieved of her duties as main nurse by Miss Rae, who was on vacation.) (The following statement was made on October 25, when Lieutenant Aspy returned to Camp Crane and Dr. J. W. Leckie assumed the role of the camp's physician.

The four-ward hospital was prepared to receive patients on October 12th. Although the shortage of nurses was to blame for the delay in establishing the hospital, the opening was held up until Wednesday because Capt. E. L. Hendricks, U.S.M.C., as the physician in charge, and Mrs. J. Pryor Williamson of Wilkes-Barre, Graduate Nurse, served as the chief nurse. The following day, on the afternoon of Wednesday, eleven male and seven female patients were received from Wilkes-Barre, Edwardsville, Plymouth, and Miner's Mills, and on Thursday, eleven female and seven male patients arrived at Wilkes-Barre, Edwardsville, Plymouth, and Miner's Mills.

In the spring of 1905, a new Emergency Hospital was established in the Pulaski School building in Dupont, Luzerne County, and in charge was visiting physician Dr. W. S. Helman of Avoca and chief nurse Miss Herman, Graduate Nurse. (On November 9, 2011, Dr. Helman was succeeded by Dr. James S. Dixon, and on November 19, 2011, Miss Herman was superseded by Miss Bessie Fadden.)

In the school building in Nanticoke, Luzerne County, the Emergency Hospital opened on October 17, with Dr. Elmer L. Hinman in charge and Miss Olwen Williams, Graduate Nurse, as the main nurse. Lieut. C. E. Yates was appointed as Dr. Hinman's replacement on October 26th, arriving in New York City that same day.

The doctors that helped out in the 5th District of Wilkes-Barrère on October 17 were medical students at the University of Buffalo, Messrs. J. A. Post and W. R. Stewart. Dr. Corrigan moved Mr. Stewart to the Wanamie Hospital, where he assisted Mr. Post. Mr. Post, in turn, was assigned to the Exeter Hospital, and then to the Plains Emergency Hospital.

Two Army Surgeons arrived at Wilkes-Bargate at the same time, with this day's arrivals listed in parentheses: Captain's Davenport and Danforth were assigned to work at Jeddo, while Captains Brown and Wroth had been reassigned to Cranberry and Lattimer, respectively. In other words, they were ordered to return to Camp Crane, Allentown on October 19th.

Spanish Flu 1918, Deadlier Than Covid-19

General Dougherty, the Chairman, presided over the meeting on October 18th, which was attended by many members of the General Committee. The hospital noted that only patients who couldn't get appropriate home care should be transported to the hospitals. He pointed out the dire scarcity of doctors and nurses in the area, and implored Nellie G. Loftus, the state nurse in charge of nurses in this section, to give her assessment of the current state of affairs. In making this point, she introduced the fact that there were thirty graduate nurses working in the 5th District who were unable to work because of illness. Another fifty graduate nurses might and should be placed in duty immediately, in addition to the eleven practical nurses.

The motion then moved: Mr. W. C. Shepherd moved that.

"The essence of this conference is that everyone, including patriotic people, would use their abilities and resources to their maximum extent to benefit the community as a whole. They are in service to their country and have a patriotic duty to carry out their service at this momentous time."

Chairman Percy A. Brown indicated that the region in Luzerne County had been divided into forty sub-districts, and that he had set up an organization in each of them. He was already aware of thirty-two of the forty organizations' reports. To help those around him from becoming infected with the flu, he proposed that pamphlets be created in numerous different languages with easy-to-follow recommendations for flu prevention and sick care.

This initiative was carried out and a six-page brochure on the subject was issued in English, Italian, and three other languages.

Mr. Brown also proposed a fund in which money could be drawn to cover the salary of a sanitary and health inspector for each sub-district.

After obtaining statistics from many significant coal-mining enterprises, Esq. Anthony Campbell said that as many as 30,000 tons of coal may have been lost to the industry because of the virus.

On proposal of Mr. W. C. Shepherd, it was voted that all districts in this district should petition all localities to form health committee committees that will use

Spanish Flu 1918, Deadlier Than Covid-19

the state's supported or recommended plan. This motion was approved, and so the chairman appointed the following individuals to the Ways and Means Committee: William C. Shepherd, Dr. Charles H. Miner, Dr. S. P. Mengel, Dr. E. L. Meyers, A. C. Campbell, and Percy A. Brown, who were tasked with creating a plan to serve as a reference for the many communities in this matter.

Walter Davis' petition to use systematic treatment for patients with flu was granted. As part of the committee, Dr. Davis, Dr. Lake, Dr. Geist, and Miss Nellie Loftus were appointed to create a plan for this systematized treatment.

Therefore, it was decided, Mr. William H. Conyngham moved to have the following voted on: "on October 26, we demand that the Chairman of the General Committee communicate by telegraph with the proper officials in Washington to notify them of our desire to keep in this community until the conditions have improved, the army doctors currently stationed here;

The Ways and Means Committee put out a proposal on October 20 during a meeting of the General and District Chairmen, during which they also shared their ideas for organizing outlying areas. Immediately after the new plan was made public, orders were given to print and disseminate it across the various villages. Fuel Conservator Campbell notified Federal Fuel Administrator Garfield that he had sent a telegram to call attention to the issue of using military doctors here so they might remain at the hospital, and Garfield ordered the army doctors to stay.

The next action was as follows:

INVENTORY OF COMMUNITY ORGANIZATION PREPARED IN THE CASE OF THE EPIDEMIC EMERGENCY.

Is the head of the community (President of the Board of Health).
The Executive Committee, which includes the Board of Health, consists of: John Burgess, as well as a representative from the Borough or Township Council.
The union appointed a representative for mine administration and my supervisor, and we're working together.
Head of a school.

volunteer with the Red Cross
National Defense Council member
Clergyman.
outstanding citizen
Will mostly work in an advisory capacity as a local physician.
Executive Emergency Evacuation Station.
is what they do
Bureau of Nursing
Publicity Bureau.
Miscellaneous.

That time, in some areas of Luzerne County, the influenza and pneumonia conditions were "terrible." Unfortunately, at Glen Lyon as well as in Wilkes-Barre Township, the matter was far more dire. Wilkes-Barre is reporting an average of around 75 new cases every day, with all the emergency facilities in the District unable to provide adequate assistance.

While conditions in Glen Lyon, Nanticoke, Wanamie, and other towns in the 5th District were in a state of "desperation," fresh cases in Wilkes-Barre numbered 120 on October 22. This date marks the first of multiple instances in which Dr. Miner and the Chairman of the General Committee received a similar communication, which was then relayed to emergency response organizations in the 5th District.

The 20th of October, 1918.

"The Commissioner of Health of Pennsylvania wrote this letter on June 5, 2013.

"To all those concerned with the issue of administering nursing to the influenza epidemic.

"a set of instructions detailing the structure of the organization (General Order No. 2.)

Until now, we have not realized that the current health crisis is causing the greatest need, and we are now in the midst of a critical shortage of trained nurses. As a result, it is imperative that we establish a plan that can be adjusted to any situation, as additional communities get involved in the crisis.

"Graduate nurses should be utilized in a way that helps the most people. This may be done by first summoning all the partially trained attendants, Red Cross employees, and finally the lay helpers. Once these students have received careful instruction in the basics of patient care, protecting themselves, and keeping infection spread to a minimum, they should direct their attention to creating a daily log of their work. On the other hand, students who will be involved in home health work will have to make a rapid traverse of the territory, supervising the work of their subordinates, instructing these subordinates, and keeping tabs on their progress. Nurses or lay aids detailed to small groups of patients, with the graduate in charge, should be used when a graduate is assigned to a hospital. In conclusion, active graduates and subordinates who follow orders and use military precision attain results that cannot be obtained by attempting to provide trained nurses to individual families or by going through the process of training many nurses in a short period of time.

"It is absolutely essential that the lives and health of doctors, nurses, and orderlies be conserved for the huge number of patients that need their services. As a result, a system should be established that distributes the time and labor of all workers evenly, according to the type of work they do. All infection prevention measures must be maintained at all times, e.g. the wearing of long gowns that cover the entire body, and the construction of surgical masks which are created from eight layers of gauze or two layers of butter cloth, and which have an 8-layer gauze head covering that covers the convex surface of a wire tea-strainer that is approximately four inches in diameter, which is then molded to fit the face from above the tip of the nose to below the point of the chin and is fastened to the head by tape

To save time and ensure accuracy, strict military discipline is required. This means that every personal preference, no matter how trivial, must be placed in service of the greater good. Leaders should show discretion in giving directions to subordinates, avoiding any task that is unnecessary or redundant. Following their supervisors' directions without hesitation or disagreement is a key subordinate responsibility. Courtesy at all times will help us attain our goal—the detection, if possible, of this major public tragedy and its deleterious effects, as well as reducing the damage and casualties it causes.

"To request assistance from an afflicted community, approach the local Department of Health official and ask who is in charge of the emergency district in which the person lives. Calls for doctors, nurses, aides, and other types of relief are included in this category. All such needs will be met as quickly as possible. To be absolutely sure, however, wherever these are available, they should be procured locally.

"The tent hospital, where patients can enjoy fresh air for 24 hours, and get sunlight from being pulled out of the hospital's grounds during the day, is the ideal emergency hospital. The wooden shacks and lean-tos like those used in T.B. treatment is excellent. Due to the lack of available window space, balconies and porches should not be used for buildings without them. When it comes to schools, open-air schools are nearly ideal; alongside them are modern schools with big grounds. Visitors should be prohibited, save for immediate family members of people who are at the end of their lives, who should wear masks and gowns.

"Invite those who wish to do something for the victims but who cannot provide medical assistance to produce protective clothing, masks, and other supplies, as well as nutritious meals such as broths or bouillon. When families are suffering, traveling kitchens or food provided by motor vehicles are quite helpful. A committee to investigate and remedy hardship should be constituted in a county. Members of this committee could help workers keep their jobs.

"All current agencies (city governments, nonprofit organizations, organizations, and societies) should be coordinated to help eliminate uncertainty and misunderstanding, as well as unnecessary expense and duplication of instructions.

"Each district is headed by a physician who serves as the district leader, who may include multiple counties in the district. The supervisor of the district is also a supervising nurse, and her district headquarters will be somewhere close to the District Chief's unless an unexpected change occurs. These two officers, representatives of the Medical and Nursing services, are all other department officers subordinate. Supervising nurses, district chiefs, and county inspectors at the epidemic headquarters are obliged to provide reports on a daily basis beginning at 1 p.m. This group of officers should ensure that all of their district subordinates have reported to them prior to this time.

It is important to keep in mind that District Chiefs and Supervising Nurses (the heads of the nursing stations within an area) are solely accountable for their district and cannot be relieved from one locality for an extended period of time. They will respond based on needs that occur, as well as department requirements.

"Bernard Royer.

"Acting Health Commissioner."

On October 23, in Plains, Luzerne County, the Maffett Street School building became the home of the eighth Emergency Hospital, with Miss May Conlon, Graduate Nurse, in charge as the hospital's main nurse.

The following United States Army medical officer, who had been stationed in the 5th District, returned to Camp Crane, which is located in the Crane District, as ordered: LIEUTENANT C. F. BAHLER, LIEUTENANT JOSEPH GOLDSTONE, LIEUTENANT G. T. MEAD, AND LIEUTENANT JAMES ASPSY. During his stay at the Hotel Sterling, Captain Hendricks delayed for a while. Daugherty sent this telegram to Gen. Peyton C. March, Chief of Staff, U.S.A., on the aforementioned date:

We have worked methodically to combat Spanish Influenza in Luzerne County, where 350,000 people reside. According to the count, 300 doctors were registered in the county, and 115 of them had volunteered for military service. In Addition to the standard hospitals, we have constructed seven emergency hospitals to deal with the additional influenza cases in the area. But three Camp Crane doctors, who went with the team, have remained. Six thousand mine workers have been diagnosed with the sickness, which means that each day the amount of anthracite coal produced by the mines has been reduced by 15,000 tons, or 300,000 tons per month. Camp Greenleaf claims that we have 4,000 military physicians in training. We will have to dispatch twenty-five physicians to this location immediately. We are experiencing an increase in the spread of the sickness, and so, medical aid is required. The doctors are completely worn out.

On October 26, Chairman Daugherty informed the commissioners of Luzerne County that the county commissioners had allocated $25,000 for fighting the virus outbreak in Luzerne County. Most committee members agreed that this money should not be distributed until the outbreak was over. However, it was said that other groups had previously made requests for funding. After further deliberation, the General Committee voted to authorize a committee consisting of the Chairman and three other committee members to create and present a strategy for spending the County's budget at a future meeting.

In early December, the City Council of Wilkes-Barre provided $5,000 in extra funding to help combat the flu outbreak in the city. In addition to the standard annual appropriation for the city's Bureau of Health, this sum was also appropriated for this year.

According to Colonel Eyer, the mortality rate at the Armory Emergency Hospital was high due to the patients' serious health problems when they arrived at the hospital. At 9:20 p.m., the Committee adjourned and went to the Lehigh Valley Railroad station, where Army medical officers who had arrived from Camp Crane in Allentown, Pennsylvania, were met. They were then assigned to their jobs and tasked with helping to prevent the spread of the flu in Luzerne County as indicated.

The State Department of Health reported that on this date, the number of patients admitted with the flu and pneumonia in hospitals in the 5th District was as follows: Hazleton Emergency, 22; Exeter Emergency, 70; Dupont Emergency, 9; Wanamie Emergency, 55; Wilkes-Barre Expression: Hazleton Emergency, 22; Exeter Emergency, 70; Dupont Emergency, 9; Wanamie Emergency, 55; Wilkes-BarrArmory Emergency, 46; Catawissa Emergency, 8; Plains Emergency, 19; Nanticoke Emergency, Hazleton State, 75; Nesbitt West Side, 14; Wyoming Valley Homeopathic, 15; Nanticoke State, 13; Mercy, 30; Wilkes-Barre State: Hazleton Emergency, 22; Exeter Emergency, 70; Dupont Emergency, 9; Wanamie Emergency, 55; Wilkes-Barre

The number of new cases reported in Luzerne County on October 28 reached 956.

The Coöperation Committee of the Greater Philadelphia Chamber of Commerce and the General Committee of the Philadelphia Area Chamber of Commerce had a joint meeting on October 28 in the chamber's offices in the Wilkes-Barré Business Building.

According to Chairman Brown, the most difficult task for the Coöperation Committee was to appreciate nurses. He further remarked that new organizations should be set up promptly in certain areas. He called for additional money for nurses, and claimed he believed more nurses could be found, with this resulting in better success in the fight against the plague.

It was voted that graduate nurses in Luzerne County should receive a salary of $120 per month, while practical nurses should earn $75 per month. The motion was approved as well, and all registered nurses were required to be under the authority of Miss Loftus and the General Committee.

It was agreed that, in all the cities, boroughs, and first-class townships in Luzerne County, every household in which influenza had spread would be informed about the disease. Furthermore, in this case, all concerns of publicity in Luzerne County about the "flu" shall be dealt with by the Chairman of the Co-op Partnership.

After this conference was adjourned, a "Publicity Bulletin" was released.

In the auditorium of the Chamber of Commerce, a meeting of all district chairmen and members of the Ways and Means Committee was convened this morning. According to reports, authorities are putting their own selfish interests above the well-being of their constituents, as well as the general health of their particular communities, by using politics as a crutch. Action will be made to have the authorities removed unless they take immediate actions to organize and protect their local communities.

In order to fight the epidemic, it was also agreed that we needed additional field nurses, and the sooner this could be done, the sooner the virus would be controlled in our area. The graduate nurses were hired at $120 per month, and the practical nurses were hired for $75 per month. Miss Nellie G. Loftus, who is stationed at the Wyoming Valley Dispensary, 184 South Washington Street, Wilkes-Barre, will be handled by all the nurses.

In addition, newspaper reports collected from residents in towns and boroughs are inaccurate, and that is unfair to the residents of these towns and boroughs. Estimates that first showed thirteen deaths in one village were in error. The true number of deaths was only three. Thus, it was determined that the Coöperation Committee's chairman would be the only person authorized to send out announcements on behalf of the general committee.

Also, we recommended to city, township, and borough officials in Luzerne County that all homes be labeled with information about the presence of influenza.

P.A.B."

Coöperation Committee chairman

This shows a drop in the number of new cases, but no decrease in the number of deaths.

Seventy-three new cases were reported on November 4 in Wilkes-Barre, and it seemed that the epidemic was almost finished in much of Luzerne County. Based on the virus, it was anticipated that about 10,000 coal miners in the county were out of work.

The General Committee meeting on November 6th, presided over by Chairman Daugherty, was fully attended in the auditorium of the Wilkes-Barre Chamber of Commerce that evening. Berwick in Columbia County and Plains in Luzerne County were still having a tough time dealing with the outbreak. He claimed that Nanticoke has also been affected by the disaster. Luzerne County had 249 deaths from the flu recorded in Newport Township. New cases and deaths are expected to occur for the next three or four weeks as conditions remain steady.

Luzerne County had been the salvation of the entire county due to the wonderful work of the countywide organization. In absence of this vaccine, the mortality rate would have been significantly higher, and many towns and neighborhoods would have experienced the full impact of the epidemic. He read a communication that had just arrived from the acting commissioner of health, which began as follows:

Efforts to end the pandemic of influenza should be made as soon as possible. If the only institutions open during the outbreak are churches and schools, care should be taken when limitations are lifted." During this perilous period, many children have been kept fully out of harm's way, and to open too soon and expose them to individuals who have recently recovered from the sickness could, in addition, reinfect the rest of the population, especially young children.

Also, as many as 25,000 public, private, and parochial school instructors have been regularly practicing nursing, and they deserve a few days of rest—preferably a week—during which they are not at work.

Please give this matter some thought, and, in conjunction with the school districts, find a way to resume classes after two-thirds of the students in any district have been free of influenza for seven days. Medical and nurse supervision is preferable during the first several days after school opens.

In my opinion, school work should resume between the hours of 12 p.m. and 2 p.m. on weekdays, and on Sundays at 8 a.m. or earlier. This is a way to gradually draw kids together and prevent the risk of overcrowding that occurs in Sunday schools if these were the first Sunday schools created. Many, especially urban, Sunday schools meet in buildings that are not sufficiently aired as well as other public schools.

Over 2,000 school teachers throughout the state have helped fight the outbreak.

It was on the motion of Percy A. Brown that the letter of the Acting Commissioner of Health was approved and that it was voted to make it publicly available as well as to urge all school boards and Sunday schools to delay the reopening of their schools unless they had first sought out advice from the

Boards of Health in their respective jurisdictions, learning whether the resumption of school would spark a new wave of the outbreak.

Daugherty, chatting in Harrisburg with the Acting Commissioner of Health Dr. Royer, says that Dr. Royer remarked that the organizational efforts of the county during the outbreak were "the finest in the country," and that the people of Luzerne County deserve great credit for the work they have done. During this portion of the ceremony, General Daugherty read a letter that he had just received from the Acting Commissioner, which read in part as follows:

I am exceedingly grateful for the wonderful narrative of healthcare during the emergencies, and to see how excited the public has become due to your committee's efforts. Because of this public health campaign, we've been able to save the lives of miners that we have previously spared due to the work of volunteer miners' community service has contributed to saving miners' lives The committee must not receive too much credit, so I will ensure that the press gives a large deal of credit to the people of the community.

As the Chair of the General Committee, Shepherd argued that the committee should report on the latest recommendations from the State Department of Health to all of the counties, because these would include the relaxation of the quarantine ban in those counties.

While the newest reports stated that there had been a general decrease in the sickness, Percy A. Brown, chairman of the Co-operation Committee, stated that the average number of new cases was roughly seven per day in each district, as opposed to a recent average of 10 cases per district. He informed the audience that on the following day, he expected to send out to every Luzerne County community chairman a questionnaire requesting certain information about the total number of cases and deaths that had occurred since the start of the epidemic, as well as a complete record of all of the people who have worked, volunteered, and were compensated. Later on, he said, he intended to organize a meeting among the various chairs to help reduce the risk of deadly epidemics occurring in the future.

As a member of the County Board of Supervisors, Supervisor Brown should request information on the number of children who are orphaned by the epidemic. He said that he would bring the information to Harrisburg, and if he could, he would ask the state for additional funds to care for these youngsters. He stated that he believed the state would raise the appropriation for the Mothers Pension Fund in order to help with these types of situations.

William C. Shepherd, a newspaper publisher, thought that using the statistical information as described would result in obtaining valuable information that would be used to compile a history of the disease. For future generations, he believes these facts should be recorded and preserved. Father McCabe proposed that we wait until the disease is fully stamped out before taking a census of all the various settlements. According to Dr. S. P. Mengel, taking a census too soon may lead to faulty information; in the final analysis, the data secured from a census should only include medical-authority facts, because no one else is qualified to determine whether or not a person who was diagnosed with influenza actually had it or something else.

The Schuylkill County Medical Inspector informed us about the things done in Pottsville, where numerous children had lost their parents to the virus. In his comments, he also suggested the creation of a community census and a permanent record that keeps track of everyone who contributed in the effort to combat the flu in Luzerne County.

Wilkes-Barre School Board member Dr. E. L. Meyers spoke on the exemplary work done by school teachers during the crisis and in other social movements, and advocated that the teachers and superintendents should be enlisted when a census of community conditions is taken. After all the discussion, a unanimous vote agreed to the following resolution.

Resolved: The Chairman of the Coöperation Committee is to advise the superintendents of all of the school districts in Luzerne County to make a community census, so that all towns will have the data necessary to prevent future epidemics, and to help prevent the Influenza Epidemic." A committee of physicians, designated by the chairman of the general committee, will create the questionnaires to be utilized by the school teachers when conducting the census.

Having resolved to implement this decision, Chair Dougherty formed a team that would design the proposed census questionnaire to be used by physicians, scientists, physicians' specialists, and generalists.

The Chairman stressed the importance of creating a distribution plan for the money that Wilkes-Barre City and Luzerne County provided for work on the cholera outbreak. He made special note of the fact that the General Committee had no intention of spending the money irresponsibly, but that only those expenses would be paid that each community could appropriately benefit from. To do justice to all parties, much care should be taken in devising a strategy that, when put into action, results in everyone getting an equal cut of the pie.

Following this motion, it was agreed that the Chairman of the General Committee could name a committee whose responsibility it would be to design and implement a plan for the distribution of the funds available for the purposes of hospital expenses and the relief of victims of the Influenza Epidemic in Luzerne County.

In order to determine the number of cases in each community, as well as the costs incurred by the various communities, the committee decided to gather as much information as possible on these two matters.

In response to a question asked by the County Medical Inspector, it was decided that the agreed-upon rates of pay for nurses should be given to the nurses from the moment their service begins.

Upon motion duly made, and seconded, the following gentlemen were afterwards appointed to assemble the Committee for the Distribution of Funds: Chairman Daugherty designated them in accordance with the meeting's decision. The names of these amazing American heroes include those of Charles H. Miner, Dr. Charles H. Conyngham, John O'Donnell, James M. Stack, Harry W. Ruggles, William J. Ruff, William C. Shepherd, and General Charles B. Daugherty. After a meeting of the committee, which had previously selected William C. Shepherd as Chairman, William J. Ruff as Treasurer, and L. K. Eldridge as Secretary, the committee members decided to re-organize and choose William C. Shepherd as Chairman, William J. Ruff as Treasurer, and L. K. Eldridge as Secretary.

Spanish Flu 1918, Deadlier Than Covid-19

The General Committee reached an agreement with various city, school, and church authorities, including the mayor, on November 7th, stating that it was safe to reopen saloons and barrooms on November 9th, as well as churches on November 10th, and motion picture houses, theaters, dance halls, etc., on November 11th.

The Catawissa Emergency Hospital (which had been operating out of a private property), which was created on November 5, shut down. Six physicians (including the chief), five graduate nurses, and two orderlies were present during the reported medical emergency. Out of the 39 patients that had been admitted, two people had died.

The Hazleton Emergency Hospital closed on November 8th. There were two U.S. military medical officers, five orderlies, and enlisted troops, as well as a nurse who was a graduate for five days who volunteered. When the hospital closed, Dr. J. W. Leckie was in charge. The overall number of hospital admissions was 109, with 55 pneumonia and 54 influenza. One influenza patient and 42 pneumonia patients were killed — 13 died within 24 hours after hospital admission.

On 11 November Exeter Emergency Hospital closed, the doctor responsible was Dr. James Dixon. Nine graduate nurses, three practical nurses, three voluntary nurses and for one part of the time three ordained nurses were employed. Patients with influenza were hospitalized to the number of 90 and patients with pneumonia to the number of 79 (total of 169).

The Emergency Armory Hospital Wilkes-Barré was closed on 14 November. This hospital, as mentioned above, was opened for patient receipt on 16 October, with the following staff: Capt. E. L. Hendricks, the U.S. Marine Corps, the physician in charge, Mrs. J. Pryor Williamson of Wilkes-Barré, a graduate nurse, the head nurse, 15 graduate nurses, 9 assistants and two civil clinics.

During the hospital's existence, a total of five physicians (including chief) were employed; fifteen were graduate-schools; twelve were volunteer-school nurses (three graduates, nine aids), ten were orderly and 15 were enlisted.

The preparation and serving of meals for patients and the hospital personnel was under the leadership of Mrs. E. Birney Carr, the Red Cross Canteen Service. The services of Ms. P. J. Higgins was engaged in preparing and baking the meals, and the quality and amount of food they served were beyond criticism under her skilled guidance.

An early system for the purchase of materials and supplies was launched. This system has acquired all the necessary materials and supplies, excluding food, by the Lieut. Charles A. Trein (2D Infantry Reserve Militia, Pennsylvania) acts as purchasing agent. The accounts issued were approved immediately by Col. S. E. W. Eyer and were ordered to be paid with little confusion and no complex bookkeeping system. With this approach and the participation of the responsible medical officers and graduate nurses, everything went smoothly and routinely.

Captain Hendricks was summoned for foreign deployment on 24 October to his battalion at Camp Crane, Allentown. Unfortunately he fell ill as he was going to depart Wilkes-Barré and was confined to his bed at the Hotel Sterling three days later. Lieut. Joseph Goldstone, U.S. Marine Corps, was posted to Armory Hospital by 25 October and was still in charge of the armor until 31 October, when he was also called back to Camp Crane for foreign service. For the second time, the hospital was deprived of a dedicated, conscientious and tireless worker.

On 28 October, Ms. J. Pryor Williamson, the Wilkes-Barré Red Cross worker for extended leave, who served as Armory Chief Nurse, was brought back to Washington. During her twelve days of work in the armory, she had put her knowledge of the hospital, her energy and her unfailing efforts on a work-base, which left no doubt as to her skill and sound judgment in the subjects under her management. Miss Antoinette Schofield, a graduate nurse in charge, followed Williamson competently as the nurse in charge of the armory until the hospital was closed down.

Captain Evan S. Evans, of the United States, was appointed to the hospital on 1 November and stayed in charge of the clinic until 14 Nov., when he, too, was ordered back to Camp Crane. Among his sunny personality and cheerful grin, Captain Evans made several friends with the patients and anyone with whom he came into touch.

On November 14, it was decided to close the hospital with only three patients. Therefore, two of the three patients were sent to City Hospital and one to Mercy Hospital. In Wilkes-Barré, an average of about 30 new cases of pandemic were reported each day. As a result, the Armory Hospital was left untouched for approximately two weeks, but as no new cases were received during this period, the wards were demolished and fumigated and the facility was ultimately closed to the public on 7 December.

All foodstuffs left behind on closure were evenly divided and donated to the City Hospital Wilkes-Barré, the Mercy Hospital and the Wyoming Valley Homopathic Hospital. Other items of use and value have been handed over, after adequate fumigation, to the authorities of the City of Wilkes-Barré, then under construction, for use in the City Hospital for Contagious Diseases.

The total number of patients admitted to the Armory Emergency Hospital was 192, including 132 men and 60 women. 94 of the patients were cases of pneumonia, of which 66 died. Three of them died of flu. Thirty-five people died within 24 hours of their hospital stay. On a single day, the highest number of patients admitted was 18—17 October. The greatest number of patients at the hospital on a single day was 62; seven were the greatest number of deaths on a single day; and the highest number of people on a single day was 14. 86 of the patients were under the age of 30 years.

Of the 192 patients received at EH, 102 were from Wilkes-Barré; 20 from Edwardsville; 22 from Swoyersville; 7 from Ashley; 6 from Plymouth; 5 respectively from Kingston and Mining Mills; four from Askam, Parse and Forty Fort; three from Maltby; two from Larksville, Sugar Notch, Nanticoke and Buttonwood; one from Plainsville and Dorranceton each; Of the 192 patients admitted into EHH Hospital, 102 were from Wilkes-Barré;

On 18 November the Plains emergency hospital was closed down, at which point the doctor was in command of Lieut. H. R. Lipscomb, U.S.A., and the nurse chief was Miss May Conlon, a graduate nurse. Five distinct medical staff (not more than one at any time) together with four graduate nursing staff, three practical nurses, six voluntary nurses, one medical student, three orderly staff and three males enlisted. 50 patients were admitted (31 influenza cases, 18 pneumonia cases, 1 croup case), of which 13 died – three of them within 24 hours after their admission to the hospital.

The Dupont Hospital was closed on 3 December, at which time the head physician was Dr. James S. Dixon and the head nurse was Miss Bessie Fadden, the successor on 19 November. There were four graduate nurses, five practical nurses (who worked part of the time), two medical units and a handful of Sisters of the Bernardine Order who were volunteers. One hundred and three patients, 83 influenza, and 20 pneumonia, were admitted to hospital. Twelve of these latter were killed—five of them within 24 hours of their hospital admission.

In relation to the cases of flu and pneumonia treated in several permanent hospitals in 5th District, the following information was derived from official reports to the County Medical Inspector from 1 October 1918 to 1. January 1919.

Homeopathic Hospital Wyoming Valley: Total Influenza Cases, 68; Pneumonia Cases, 55; Total Deaths, 27.

Mercy Hospital: Total influenza, 133; pneumonia, 131; total deaths, 87—including 22 deaths within twenty-four hours following their hospital admission.

City Hospital, Wilkes-Barré: Total number of cases, 457, 223 influenza cases and 234 cases of influenza-pneumonia. There were two hundred and thirty-four men, and 223 women. The total death toll was 135. Of the hospital workers, 72 were suffering from pneumonia and four were killed.

Pittston Hospital: Total influenza cases, 67 (males, 26; females, 41); cases of pneumonia, 32, 13 of which were tragically ended.

Hazleton State Hospital: Total influenza patients, 275; pneumonia patients, 216, of which 113 died.

Hospital Berwick: Total number of cases of influenza, 113; pneumonia cases, 25; total number of cases of influenza, 16.

On 18 November, influenza pneumonia cases in Wilkes-Barré were so worrying that the local governments enacted yet another quarantine order, banning all entertainment centers and restricting public assemblies. This prohibition was repealed eleven days later, despite the average daily incidence of new flu and pneumonia being approximately 35. However, the city's public schools were closed for approximately two months and only reopened on December 4th, although about 18 new influenza cases each day were reported in Wilkes-Barré. Conditions seemed to improve in other sections of the county.

On 15 December the local authorities ordered the closure of all colleges, with the exception of the City High School and the private schools of the same grade, in view of the substantial increase of influenza cases in Wilkes-Barré. Children below the age of 14 years were also prohibited from attending theaters and movie presentations, traveling by public transport, and visiting shops. Sunday school sessions should likewise be stopped. The outbreak appeared especially frequent among children.

On December 17th one hundred and four cases of influenza in Wilkes-Barré were notified and on the next day the municipal authorities imposed additional restrictions on quarantine, the main of which was to prevent the entry and leaving of people in quarantined homes, except for doctors and others with special permits.

On 19 December, the General Committee met with Wilkes-Barré, Dorranceton and Hanover health workers. Chairman Brown of the Coöperation Committee revealed that, up to that date, 2,872 influenza and pneumonia deaths had occurred in Luzerne County, with 345 in Wilkes-Barré. The County Medical Inspector reviewed the situation in the county briefly and indicated that officials do not report the genuine situations in their localities in some cases.

At a meeting of the General Committee held on 21 December, the County Medical Inspector stated that conditions were so high for different communities within 5th District that, except where requested by the authorities of their respective communities, the Interim Commissioner of the State Department of Health was not willing to order a further quarantine ban. Dr. Clark of Wilkes-Health Barré's Bureau indicated that the situation in the town had been better in the past four days than it was some time ago—only 35 new cases had been registered. He claimed that 1,020 cases had been reported so far this month, while only 825 cases had been reported in November. The disease attacks more youngsters and fewer adults.

Mayor Kosek said he was against paralyzing the community's business, but he felt that everything necessary should be done to end the disease. He stated that he was in support of promoting the matter and requested officials in the surrounding villages to collaborate on regulatory enforcement with the city authorities.

The resolutions were then adopted to enforce rigorously any subsequent epidemic fighting plans that would have to be put into effect until all the danger had gone; to close children's entertainment areas; and to avoid public funerals and overcrowding at public gatherings. Dr. S. P. Mengel then adopted the following resolution unanimously:

It is settled that this committee supports the rules and regulations adopted by the Health Board of the City of Wilkes-Barré and that we call for its strict enforcement and we commit ourselves to cooperation with the authorities to bring it to fruition; and also we call on all the public and the officials of all of Luzerne County communities to cooperate in the implementation of this directive.

On 23 December Major Kosek of the city of Wilkes-Barré announced officially that, if the city's public did not voluntarily comply with the reasonable quarantine regulations, he would impose the most comprehensive and absolute quarantine, regardless of what interests, which was yet ordered.

In the approaching holiday season, officers of the city's health office strongly opposed the lifting of the prohibition on public dances, cabarets, Sunday School sessions and other public meetings. On 1 January 1919, however, the ban on moving houses was withdrawn and the remaining quarantine limits were abolished on 10th of the month, and the Sunday schools and public and private schools in the town continued.

Soup was delivered to the neighboring Wilkes-Barré neighborhoods and sent to the apartments of the visiting nurses and to the Friendless Children's Home. Corresponding numbers of desserts have been supplied to the outskirts and the Friendly Children's Home in Wilkes-Barré. In great quantities, jellies and marmalades were given and supplied with soup and desserts. The sum of $500.00 was provided to influenza patients for free milk.

Although the Canteen had been on troop trains during the month of December, the work continued incidentally to the outbreak. Large amounts of soup, custard and milk from the Canteen Headquarters were provided to people and families in and around the city. There were served three thousand nine hundred seventy-four persons. The soup distributed two thousand four hundred and fifty-six quarts; 167 quarts, corresponding custard portions, had been sent into Georgetown, and 1312 quarts to the apartments of the visiting nurses. Eight hundred five quarters of milk have been distributed. Two hundred and three lunches were packed at the affected households with volunteer nurses on duty. On Christmas Day, twenty-four quarters of ice cream were delivered. Desserts have been distributed using the following: 739 milk quarters, 84 quartz gelatins, 11712 twelve eggs, 1012 twelve lemons, 4 quarters of vanilla, 47 cornstarch boxes, 53 tapioca boxes, 33 gelatin boxes, 12 jello lemon boxes, 85 pound of sugar.

On 10 December 1918 at a meeting of the Greater Wilkes-Barré Chamber of Commerce with the Chairman, Philip R. Bevan and the Minister, Hayden Williams in charge, we had a very thorough discussion with regard to the large number of children who had been orphaned by the flu scourge in Lucerne County (2,390, as noted on page —n?, ante). The following resolution was adopted as follows:

"Resolved to create a committee to examine this question and offer suggestions at a forthcoming Chamber meeting."

Spanish Flu 1918, Deadlier Than Covid-19

The following Committee was formed by President Bevan: William C. Shepherd, Chair; Percy A. Brown, C. F. Brisbin, John N. Conyngham, Charles E. Clift, William H. Conyngham, Fuller R. This Committee convened on 3 January 1919 and after careful debate, unanimously held that it would be essential to organize a general committee from various regions of the County of Lucerne before any attention could be given to a specific Plan for the permanent relief of influenza orphans. President Shepherd has said that any relief plan should be adopted for the entire county. He also suggested that it should be decided whether existing charitable organizations can or should not take care of any one of the children or whether a special institution should be founded.

Mr. Hendershot and others present raised the issue of whether the Mothers' Pension Fund could handle any one of the children. It was acknowledged that if this were done, the Funds should be increased. Since some counties of the State do not have such a fund, it was suggested that the local council might achieve an increase in its resources from the government money not drawn from other countries entitled to the fund.

Mr Brisbin informed me of the investigation then under his leadership of representatives of the Red Cross and others to ascertain the conditions surrounding the epidemic. He stated that when the inquiries were concluded, there was definite information within two or three weeks on the exact number of orphans to be permanently provided for. He noted that in many circumstances, orphans are placed under the care of family or other people, and that ultimately, the number of orphans provided by the general public is not as high as expected.

It was then decided that a committee, the representative of the whole county, should be established on Mr. Brown's motion:

"Plans for the permanent relief of all orphans in need of flu are to be developed, with a view to securing information on permanent relief plans for those cities before this general committee meeting, which is to be held on 20 January 1919, the Secretary should communicate to the various Cities of Pennsylvania and other States where the epidemic was serious."

Spanish Flu 1918, Deadlier Than Covid-19

In keeping with this resolution, it was determined that the following persons should be asked to meet with the Chamber of Commerce on 20 January 1919 at 3 p.m. to establish a "permanent influenza orphan assistance organization" in Luzerne County. Ms. William C. Shepherd, Mr. Percy A. Brown, Mr. F. Brisbin, Mr. William H. Conyngham, Mr. John N. Conyngham, Mr. John D. Farnham, Ms. J. M. Huber, Ms. Mary Brady, Ms. Charles H. Miner, Ms. S. P. Mengel, Mrs. Eugene W. Mulligan, Mrs. George Galland, Mrs. Francis A. Phelps, Ms. Andrew Hobart, Mrs. Nellie Ritchie, Mrs. Mulligan, Mrs. Francis A. Phelps, Ms.

In reaction to the reports given to the stated people, some thirty-five of them were assembled in the afternoon of January 20, 1919 in the auditorium of the Chamber of Commerce Wilkes-Barré. Mr. John N. Conyngham acted as Chairman Pro Tem at the request of President Shepherd. Then Mr Shepherd described the aim of the gathering and the need to provide an adequate way to care for children in the county who were left in an impoverished state via the influenza pandemic.

The pro-tem Chairman inquired if a permanent organization should be constituted or not. Mr. Mulhall considered it wise to operate through some existing body and to have the authority to enforce any legislation relevant to the situation. He offered United Charities as such and in addition to that recommendation, Mr Schmoll reported that the United Charities of Hazleton took care of 46 influenza orphans at that time.

The president of the Mothers' Pension Fund, Mrs Galland, believes that the greatest approach would be to leave as many children to their surviving parents as possible and that virtually every situation could be dealt with by the Pension Fund - if appropriations were substantially raised for it.

On Rev. Mr. Haynes' proposal, it was finally voted that a temporary body, called the Chamber of Commerce's Committee of Cooperation, should be established to cooperate with existing agencies on inquiry and remedy for all meritorious situations.

Mr Brisbin, Chairman of the Civilian Relief Department of the Red Cross Wyoming Valley Chapter, said his Department has launched investigations by other committees or organizations regardless of any arrangement that had been or should be reached. In the same line as in the case of the Red Cross the Women's Committee of the Council of National Defense was said, Mr. Brisbin pointed out that there was a potential of major confusion and complications as a result of the overlap.

Mrs Phelps and Miss Brady (last employee of the United Charities of Wilkes-Barré) spoke about conditions found in many homes that reigned in poverty and where something had to be done to protect these families, because landlords were unable to pay their rents, from being expelled from the homes of the families. Mr Mulhall then enquired why the poor boards could not, in poor circumstances, pay the rents of households. Mr Dodson indicated that while the Poor Board of the Central District was not in favor of paying rent publicly, he thought it would silently take care of the rent by paying the United Charities with money to do so. Mr. Farnham said the Red Cross has some money to use for this purpose.

On Mr. Hendershot's suggestion, a committee was then elected to work in collaboration with the State Department of Health in an attempt to get financial assistance for all influenza orphans from the State Legislature. Thus Fuller R. Hendershot, John D. Farnham and Percy A. Brown were appointed by the Chairman.

On Mr Haynes' motion, it was then adopted that an immediate plan for permanent relief of influenza victims should be delayed until 22 January. This meeting should be attended by the Secretary, who should invite representatives of the Red Cross, the United Charities and the Poor Councils of Lucerne and Carbon Counties.

About 20 participants attended the delayed meeting of the Committee for Cooperation of the Chamber of Commerce on 22 January 1919. The President was Mr William C. Shepherd and the secretary was L. K. Eldridge. Mr. Shepherd remarked that it was the consensus that all orphans should, as far as practicable, be retained in each other's homes or cared for by family or friends. Mr. Brisbin reviewed the operations of the Civilian Relief of the Red Cross Department, indicating that case investigations were taking place and that the county, in its view, had sufficient organizations to take care of the task, but that money was very needed.

Mr. Hendershot then requested the appointment of a committee to speak with the Poor Council, the Red Cross and other organisations, to raise funds for relief operations. After this motion was put into effect, the Chairman named William H. Conyngham (Chairman), Dr. Charles H. Miner, Anthony C. Campbell, Harold N. Rust, and Rev. Selden L. Haynes, to the following committee, which would be known as the Ways and Means Committee.

Then, Charles E. Keck, Q.S., Solicitor for the Central District Poor Board, reviewed the tasks and restrictions of the Central District Board, and said that its members would be happy to meet with the newly designated committee and discuss funding for relief. Judge S. J. Strauss made several very prompt statements at this point, that a committee should be constituted to provide the capability and usefulness of the Wilkes-Barré Home for Friendless Children. He remarked that, in his perspective, there is no need for additional organisations, but the Committee should cooperate with current organisations.

At the meeting of the Coöperation Committee of the Chamber of Commerce on 31 January 1919 Mr. Rust reported to the Committee of Ways and Means that he conferred on the Central District Attorney's Office the Poor Committee which informed the committee that, where necessary, the Board would investigate and administer all relief.

Mr. Rust was of the opinion that this committee should take action to ensure that the Board correctly handled worthy cases, as taxpayers had made provision of funds for the Poor Board. In addition, as a rule of law prohibits the payment by the board of rents, the matter should be dealt with by the Red Cross; that close cooperation in investigation cases should take place between the Wyoming Valley Chapter of the Red Cross and the Poor Committee of the Central District; that immediate relief, where necessary, should be provided; and that the disbursement should be granted, if necessary; Mr. Farnham stated that, in his opinion, as far as they went, the Red Cross money will be available.

On Mr Rust's request, it was decided that the Civil Relief Department of the Red Cross Valley Chapter should take the fifty special cases to the Poor Committee of the Central District; that those cases should be checked against the Central Poor District relievers; and, that it be determined that there are persons who do not receive reliable aid.

On Mr. Conyngham's proposal it was approved to ask the Poor Committee to employ as many experienced women as possible to investigate and look after situations following the withdrawal of the Red Cross and other organizations. Rev. Dr. Farr advised that the Coöperation Committee should get a comprehensive and final report from Mr. Brisbin on the major work done by the Red Cross Civilian Relief Committee, which was led and managed by Mr. Brisbin, and was briefly referred to here before. There were no additional transactions, the committee postponed sine die.

A detailed report on the operations of the Civilian Relief Committee is to be found in "The History of the American Red Cross Wyoming Valley Chapter," which will be published shortly.

The Committee for the Distribution of Funds for Influenza Victims Care and Relief, whose appointment is previously reported, held several business meetings related to its obligations. The discussions were thoroughly held during a meeting on 21 March 1919 concerning the various emergency hospitals, following which Mr. Conyngham urged that all the General Committee bills be paid at once. This motion has been adopted. Mr. Hendershot then requested that the treasurer pay the amounts of the individual emergency hospital bills approved by the Committee. This motion has been adopted.

This committee accepted the following rules of procedure for the settlement of bills arising from the creation of the seven emergency hospitals in County Luzerne at a following meeting unanimously:

(1) The fact that checked bills should be paid for the construction of the buildings or the alteration or installation of temporary hospitals.

'(2) The confirmed bills on everyday maintenance – food, drugs, medicine, overhead expenses of light and fuel – shall be approved and paid, coupled with the special costs approved by the General Committee for the activity of the general organization in the County.

(3) Bills for established hospitals and bills for regular hospitals and charities, as well as for the work of staff in isolated households, cannot be approved and paid as appropriations for the specific purpose of setting up or maintaining the hospitals in this work were appropriated for this epidemic.'

The Distribution Committee met on 4 April 1919 and decided to produce a "Letter of information on the activity of the Distribution Committee." This letter was then written with a short summary of the organisation, the activities it had carried out, and was formally disseminated when it was signed by the members of the committee. Extracts from this letter are as follows:

"The appropriation of monies by the County of Lucerne was made by an Act of the Legislature of Pennsylvania enacted on 14 May 1915 and partially read as follows:

"'Part 1 * * * The County Commissioners of any county may make money available for the support of any hospital within the bounds or without that county which carries out charity activities and gives treatment and medical care to the citizens of that county.

"'Section 2. All acts and portions in breach of this Act will be abolished.'

"The members of the City Council made the Wilkes-Barré allocation by means of a resolution reading as follows:

"It is vital that the equipment and upkeep of the Armory Emergency Hospital are needed to combat the influenza epidemic and that much equipment is to be afterwards employed in the Wilkes-Barré City Emergency Contagious Disease Hospital, which is nearly finished.

That, therefore, it be decided, that $5,000 or so much of the City of Wilkes-Barré should be allocated to equipment and maintenance of the armoury or other hospital; that the Citizens' Board responsible should submit a bill, properly audited, to the City of Wilkes-Barré; and that the City pay these bills in the amount of an appropriation approved; and that the equipment should be whickened.

www.ingramcontent.com/pod-product-compliance
Lightning Source LLC
Chambersburg PA
CBHW070140230526
45472CB00004B/1612